Michael Donald Misfeldt

Dealing with Suicide & Depression

Getting Out of the Pit

Copyright © 2024 by Michael Donald Misfeldt.

All rights reserved. No part of this publication may be reproduced, distributed, or transmitted in any form or by any electronic or mechanical means, including information storage and retrieval systems, without a prior written permission from the publisher, except by reviewers, who may quote brief passages in a review, and certain other noncommercial uses permitted by the copyright law.

Library of Congress Control Number: 2024923105

ISBN: 979-8-89228-269-7   (Paperback)
ISBN: 979-8-89228-270-3   (Hardcover)
ISBN: 979-8-89228-271-0   (eBook)

Printed in the United States of America

DEDICATION

This book is dedicated to the incredible people who have walked alongside me in my journey, offering inspiration, strength, and hope.

To my mother, Neva, and father, Donald, whose love and guidance shaped who I am.

To my aunt, Lorena, and my stepmother, Edith, for their nurturing spirits.

To my children, Melissa, Michael Jr., and Michelle, for being the light that keeps me going.

To my pastors, Eddie Diaz, Eric Thomas, Mark Lebsack, Tim Nellis, Matt Doan, Ron Rogalski, Jim McCarty, and John Sherman—thank you for your wisdom, compassion, and unwavering support. You've helped me find faith in the darkest times.

To the men in the various groups and Bible studies, your fellowship has been a source of strength and encouragement. You've shown me the power of community and vulnerability.

A special thank you to my psychologist, Daniel Nunez, for your invaluable insights and care. Your guidance has been a cornerstone of my healing.

And to all those who have stood beside me—your presence in my life has been a gift beyond measure.

HISTORY OF DEPRESSION & SUICIDE or GETTING OUT OF THE PIT

Introduction

Life can be unpredictable, often throwing us into valleys of despair that seem too deep to escape. For many, depression feels like a shadow that blocks out all light, a silent struggle that isolates us from hope, joy, and even from the people we love. I know this feeling all too well because I've been there. This book is a journey through my darkest moments, the weight of depression, and the suicidal thoughts that often felt too heavy to bear. But more importantly, it's a testament to the healing power of faith, resilience, and community.

I didn't walk this path alone. Even when I felt abandoned, there was a guiding light—one that came not from me but from God. My journey through depression is intertwined with my spiritual journey, one that taught me valuable lessons about love, forgiveness, and grace. It's this combination of personal experience and spiritual reflection that I hope will offer you, the reader, both comfort and practical tools for your own healing.

In this book, I will share my personal story—the challenges of growing up in a military family, dealing with feelings of inadequacy, navigating relationships, and the loss of loved ones. I will also explore the depths of depression, my attempts to end my life, and how I found a way back to living with purpose and hope.

You'll find not only my story but also spiritual insights, practical advice, and biblical truths that I discovered along the way. Whether you're struggling with depression, supporting a loved one, or simply seeking deeper spiritual understanding, this book is for you.

The journey from darkness to dawn isn't easy, and I won't pretend that it is. But it's a journey worth taking. There is hope, even in the most difficult moments. And while the light might seem faint at first, it's there—waiting for you to take the next step.

Let this book be a guide, a companion, and a source of comfort as you navigate your own valleys and peaks. Together, let's walk from darkness into the light of dawn.

Childhood and Early Years

I grew up in a military family, always on the move. My younger brother was born two years after me, and I remember the story of how our mom almost died giving birth to him. That was a tough start for our family.

Dad was a perfectionist, raised by a strict father and a loving mother on a farm in Minnesota. He had four siblings, one of whom, my uncle, became an art professor at Bowling Green University and remained single, choosing to travel extensively in Europe instead of settling down.

Mom, on the other hand, stayed home to raise two rambunctious boys. She struggled with obsessive-compulsive tendencies, which made it hard for her to show us affection. But looking back, I know she loved us in the best way she could.

As a military family, we moved a lot—Germany, then back to the States, then overseas again, every three years like clockwork. I made new friends wherever we went, but each time we moved, I felt like I had to start all over again. I often felt out of place and undeserving of the love and attention I craved, especially from my father, who worked for a top security agency in the Army. He was never allowed to talk about his job, and the stress of it eventually gave him ulcers. His work schedules were unpredictable, and while I know now that he loved us, it was hard to see that affection growing up.

I tried to fit in by getting involved in sports, but it never quite clicked for me. In Little League, I could never manage to hit the ball, and I often struck out or walked to first base, embarrassed and frustrated. I tried out for the baseball team in 9th grade, but I didn't make the cut—my dad was away on his last tour of duty in Vietnam at the time, which made the rejection sting even more.

In 11th grade, I decided to give track a try. I made the JV team, running the half-mile. I had some success in competitions and even joined the Cross-Country team during my senior year. Running gave me a sense of accomplishment, something to hold onto in the midst of the constant change.

My first year of college, I continued with Cross-Country at a small school where I studied Mechanical Engineering on a state scholarship. The scholarship covered tuition, but I had to work summers at a goat dairy to pay for room, board, and books. I worked hard, but by my senior year, I had to give up running to take on more work to save for college.

After graduating high school, I worked at an MG-Jaguar dealership, washing cars, picking up parts, and even delivering vehicles to customers. One of my favorite memories from that time was driving a brand-new XJ12 to Beverly Hills—it felt like a small victory. But it wasn't all smooth sailing. Once, I damaged a car while picking up parts, and I thought I'd be fired. Instead, I offered to make up for the damages in any way I could, and the owner accepted my offer to help with other tasks.

Growing up on Army bases or with other military families off-base, I lived a pretty sheltered life. My parents were strict about teaching us responsibility. If we wanted anything extra, we had to earn it. I still remember the time we lived in Ethiopia for three years. My brother and I wanted horses that the Embassy was selling, but my parents said we'd have to cover the room and board costs. So, we started delivering the *Army Times* newspaper whenever it arrived by plane. We earned $1 a month per customer, starting with 50 customers. By the time we were preparing to leave Ethiopia, we had grown that to 150 customers, which was a big deal for two young boys in 1968.

In December of my freshman year, we moved back to California, but my dad was stationed in Vietnam. My aunt and uncle lived nearby, and their youngest daughter became like the sister I never had. My dad returned from Vietnam after a year, and one of the first things he did was teach me how to drive a stick-shift car, a skill that came in handy later when I worked at a car dealership.

While my dad was away, my family attended church with my aunt and uncle. I remember responding to an altar call and accepting Jesus as my Savior, but it wasn't the experience I expected—I didn't feel warmly welcomed, almost like they thought I wasn't sincere. That left a lasting impression on me. Not long after my dad returned, we moved again, which meant starting over at a new high school for my junior and senior years.

After my dad left the Army, he worked with my uncle delivering mobile homes all over the country, so we didn't spend much time together again. Not long after, my dad developed bleeding ulcers and had to undergo surgery at the Presidio. I was part of a youth group at the time, and I asked for prayers for my dad. When he was healed, it made a profound impact on me and influenced my decision to consider going to seminary. But despite that desire, my parents persuaded me to attend college instead, and I ended up receiving a scholarship to a school in Southern California.

DEALING WITH SUICIDE & DEPRESSION

After two years, though, I dropped out of college. I had lost interest, and I was also working part-time for a trucking company during the week and weekends. Joining a fraternity didn't help my studies either, but that's where I met my future first wife at a social event. During those years, I also became close friends with a student from Tracy, California. We'd carpool home together for holidays like Thanksgiving and Christmas, and we're still good friends to this day.

My friend started working for a small trucking company after dropping out of college, and I followed suit, working part-time until I secured a full-time position as a driver. Around that time, I married my wife, who was still finishing her degree in Early Childhood Education. We made plans to wait five years before starting a family and hoped to buy a house. Her parents eventually helped us purchase a home.

Five years into our marriage, my mom was diagnosed with a brain tumor that had been misdiagnosed earlier. My daughter was only a month old when my mom passed away at the age of 52, but at least she knew she had a granddaughter. The funeral took place on my 26th birthday, a day forever etched in my memory. My mom and I had always been close, and even now, I get emotional at times when I think about her. After her death, I grew closer to my dad, and I was relieved when he found someone special later in life who brought him joy again.

I spent 24 years working at the same company, starting as a driver for the first 16 years. Eventually, I moved into the office as a Planner-Dispatcher and Assistant Manager, but later found myself back behind the wheel. I had to fast-track getting my Class A license after an office mix-up. I took responsibility for the mistake, even though someone else was partly to blame but wouldn't admit it. To get my Commercial Driver's License (CDL), I had to pass a physical. That's when I discovered just how high my blood pressure had become. The doctor refused to let me leave until my blood pressure dropped, and I was told that if I hadn't sought treatment, I would likely have had a stroke within two years. Despite feeling like it was unfair to be put back into a truck, I realize now that God was looking out for me, even when I didn't know it.

The timing of that health scare couldn't have been worse. During the six years I worked in the office, my life unraveled. I went through a divorce, filed for bankruptcy, lost my house, and my dad passed away from prostate cancer—likely due to his exposure to Agent Orange during his time in Vietnam. It all happened within a single year. Looking back, I now recognize that I was in a deep state of depression. I stopped going to the church I loved, cut off communication with my family, and buried myself in work. My schedule was brutal—4 PM to 4 AM from Sunday to Friday. I would pick up my kids after school on Fridays, and we'd spend weekends together, often going to the movies. Then, on Sundays, I'd drop them back off at their mom's house and head to work.

Once I got my blood pressure under control and renewed my Class A license, things started to shift. But two years later, our company lost its major contract with Gap stores, and we ended up closing and selling the business. Thankfully, with my CDL, I found another job fairly quickly, though no company could match the salary I had been earning in the office. As a thank you for 20 years of service, my old company gave me a gift—a cruise for two. I waited a year and decided to use it to take my three kids on an Alaskan cruise.

My daughters were 18 and 14, and my son was 16. We spent seven days cruising the Inside Passage, but I couldn't really relax until we reached Vancouver and boarded the ship. My oldest daughter didn't make any new friends on board, so we ended up spending a lot of quality time together. Sometimes, people gave us strange looks, mistaking us for a couple, but we didn't mind. We made the most of our trip, doing things like taking a floatplane to a cabin across from a glacier for a salmon bake, biking around Valdez, and kayaking. It was one of the best vacations of my life, even though I was still struggling with depression and hadn't done anything about it. But, as always, God had other plans for me.

DEALING WITH SUICIDE & DEPRESSION

I had planned to visit my aunt and uncle in Anchorage after the cruise, but a month before we left, they told me they'd be in California for the entire month of August. So, I decided to cut the trip short by a day and fly home instead of staying overnight. The catch was that 3,000 bikers and their support crews were leaving Anchorage on the same day. The ticket agent could only get us seats on a later flight, but we couldn't sit together. I told her that was fine—my daughters were old enough to manage on their own, and my son and I would sit together.

On the flight from Anchorage to Los Angeles, my son took the middle seat, and I sat on the aisle. A woman sat by the window wearing a t-shirt from an AIDS research fundraiser, so I immediately assumed she was gay. As we talked during the four-hour flight, I shared parts of my story, and she did the same. To my surprise, she wasn't gay and lived in Redondo Beach, not far from my home in Long Beach. She'd been on the trip hoping to meet someone in the support crew, but it hadn't worked out. She'd never been married, and she wasn't dating anyone at the time. Before we parted ways, she invited me to visit her church.

At that point, I wasn't attending church, and I had no interest in dating anyone. My kids were teenagers, and I didn't feel like sharing them with someone new after everything we'd been through with the divorce. But something nudged me to visit her church anyway. I arrived a half-hour early, and she was running late. The older ladies in the congregation made sure she knew a man was waiting for her, and after the service, we went out for breakfast at a nearby restaurant. The same older ladies from church were there, trying to play matchmaker, but I wasn't interested. Yet, as I was about to say goodbye, she kissed me on the cheek. That caught my attention.

We started dating and eventually married a year and a half later. My kids were part of the ceremony, and even my stepmom, brother, his wife, and my former pastor came. I reconciled with my family, largely thanks to the encouragement of my new wife. After our Alaska trip and some time dating, I met her family, who lived in Torrance, not far from where I lived. It turns out I already knew her mother—I used to see her every day at Western Airlines, where she worked in the freight department. It's amazing how God brought two broken people together when we needed each other most.

We got married in May 2003, and I started a new job as a Class A driver just a month earlier, in April. As a regional driver, I would come home every other day, but it wasn't an ideal start to our marriage. I'd leave before my wife got home, and I'd come back after she'd already left for work. Thankfully, after three months, I was able to transfer to a different project, and I started coming home almost every night. It was a relief, and we began attending a church in Anaheim Hills. We liked the pastor, who we'd met during an Engaged Encounter retreat before we got married. One of the most amazing things we experienced was introducing each other to our families. Not a single person objected to our relationship. I don't know if it was because we were older or because God was bringing two very different families together in a way that only He could.

Looking back at my career, after working at the same pastor we met attending an Engaged Encounter before getting married. One of the amazing things we encountered me introducing each other to the families there as not one person who had an objection to either of us, maybe it was because we were older or God bringing two different families from two completely different backgrounds.

After working for the same company now for 21 years I have been through multiple job positions and responsibilities that seemed like disappointments or setbacks when they happen they are really just preparing you for new challenges to overcome or new opportunities to develop new skills for what God has planned for you all along if only we could see the Big Picture instead of being focused on the present circumstance which I have to say honestly I haven't always handled well by letting my ego focusing on what I think is the correct action that should be taken. If we would only look at life as playing on a baseball team that is concentrating on being the best and putting the right players on the field at the right time. Is there any other sport where someone is celebrated when they don't even bat at 50% or so much of the time their performance is structured by minute details. I've had the opportunity to be a Trainer, Mentor, Safety Coordinator, Instructor, Safety Supervisor, and a Driver and had the good fortune to make a honest living to support my family, help raise three wonderful and gifted children int being productive adults, worship ny God and learn more about him every day despite my failures, hangups or fears. I am truly blessed beyond my deepest desires and during my bouts of depression I have attempted suicide twice by taking pain pills and not planning on waking up thinking I was going to escape whatever pain I was feeling or though: I was beyond help or usefulness and really didn't love himself even though I know God loves me for who I am despite my attempts to hide from him and not accept his grace. It got to the point where I stopped taking all of my medications for high blood pressure, diabetes, high cholesterol, etc. as I was slowly trying to give up on life altogether but I received a call from my primary doctor that she wanted to see me the next day to go over same medical issues, it normally takes at least two months to get an appointment to see her but I think God instructed her to call me. I have since got back on all of my medications, recovered from secondary polycythemia because my body was producing too many red blood cells causing headaches, dizziness, fatigue and chest pains got my sleep apnea under control and passed a DOT physical to continue driving.

Just recently I was driving to work and my car acted like it was running out of fuel which was weird because I had just filled up the tank, I was able to coast to the side of the freeway shoulder to avoid traffic, after trying several times to restart the car and was unsuccessful I called off work ard called AAA who sent out a tow truck but could only get me off the freeway as his shift was almost over and as it turned out he had to go hone and take his kids to school, after getting me off the freeway he offered to see if he could start the car, after I checked to make sure the car wasn't overheating and the oil was good I said sure it couldn't hurt to try, and it started right up, so I cancelled the tow and drove home, but my wife convinced me to go to the mechanic and get it checked out, it turns out the fuel line on my 2006

Nissan Altima was brittle and leaking fuel which could have caused an engine fire and poss bly ignited into flames, I feel that God was watching over me and providing his protection once again, even if you don't believe in God its to hard to believe all these events are just coincidence.

MICHAEL D MISFELDT

05/04/2024

THE THOUGHTS AND EMOTIONS SERIES

WHAT IS GOD'S HEART ON
DEPRESSION?

Excerpt from
KEYS FOR LIVING LIBRARY

DEPRESSION
Walking from Darkness into the Dawn

What Is God's Heart on Depression?

The pressures and stresses of life often weigh us down. When our hearts are heavy and our heads are low, the clouds of depression seem to block out any ray of hope. But even in our depression, God walks with us, carries our burdens, and shines the light of His Word on our despair.

> *"The LORD is God, and he has made his light shine on us."*
> (PSALM 118:27)

God is with us in our depression.
"Do not fear, for I am with you; do not be dismayed, for I am your God. I will strengthen you and help you; I will uphold you with my righteous right hand" (ISAIAH 41:10).

> *"Even in our depression, God walks with us, carries our burdens, and shines the light of His Word on our despair."*

God sees our pain and suffering.
"God, see the trouble of the afflicted; you consider their grief and take it in hand" (PSALM 10:14).

God hears our cries and listens to us in our pain.
"... the LORD has heard my weeping" (PSALM 6:8).

God wants to give us light in our darkness.
"It is you who light my lamp; the LORD my God lightens my darkness" (PSALM 18:28 ESV).

DEALING WITH SUICIDE & DEPRESSION

God wants to lift us up when we're feeling down.
"The LORD upholds all who fall and lifts up all who are bowed down" (PSALM 145:14).

God wants us to talk to Him when we're depressed.
"Trust in him at all times, you people; pour out your hearts to him, for God is our refuge" (PSALM 62:8).

God wants to comfort us.
"I, yes I, am the one who comforts you" (ISAIAH 51:12).

God wants to give us peace.
"Peace I leave with you; my peace I give you. I do not give to you as the world gives. Do not let your hearts be troubled and do not be afraid" (JOHN 14:27).

God wants to give us hope.
"For I know the plans I have for you,' declares the LORD, 'plans to prosper you and not to harm you, plans to give you hope and a future'" (JEREMIAH 29:11).

God wants us to trust Him.
"The LORD is my strength and my shield; my heart trusts in him, and he helps me" (PSALM 28:7).

God wants us to comfort others who are depressed.
"The Father of compassion and the God of all comfort . . . comforts us in all our troubles, so that we can comfort those in any trouble with the comfort we ourselves receive from God" (2 Corinthians 1:3–4).

God will one day wipe away all our tears—and there will be no more sorrow or suffering.
"He will wipe every tear from their eyes, and there will be no more death or sorrow or crying or pain. All these things are gone forever" (Revelation 21:4 NLT).

Symptoms of Depression

The American Psychiatric Association's (APA) *Diagnostic and Statistical Manual of Mental Disorders,* 5th ed. (DSM-5) lists nine key symptoms of depression. It says that a person must have at least five of the following symptoms, lasting two weeks or longer, to be considered a major depressive episode. At least one of the five symptoms must be either persistent sadness or loss of interest.

- Persistent feelings of sadness, anxiousness, or "emptiness" most or all of the time
- Complete or near complete loss of interest or pleasure in activities that were once enjoyable
- Significant change in appetite or weight
- Difficulty sleeping most nights or sleeping too much
- Agitated thoughts and movements (i.e., fidgeting, pacing, tapping fingers or feet) or slowed responses
- (i.e., pausing more when talking; speaking slower, more quietly, or infrequently; moving slowly)
- Chronically fatigued, easily decreased energy
- Feelings of worthlessness or disappointment in oneself
- Lack of concentration, focus, memory retention, or inability to make decisions
- Recurring thoughts of death or suicide or suicide attempts

Instead of diagnosing yourself with depression, first consult a mental health professional (psychiatrist, psychologist, licensed professional counselor) who can give you an educated assessment after conducting a detailed analysis of your situation and symptoms. There is no shame in reaching out for help.

The psalmist, by his own admission, reminds us just how necessary it is to admit our need for help—first to God
. . . then also to others.

DEALING WITH SUICIDE & DEPRESSION

"Be gracious to me, O LORD, for I am languishing;
heal me, O LORD, for my bones are troubled.
My soul also is greatly troubled.
But you, O LORD—how long?
Turn, O LORD, deliver my life;
save me for the sake of your steadfast love."
(PSALM 6:2–4 ESV)

Key Verse to Memorize

"Why am I so depressed? Why this turmoil within me?
Put your hope in God, for I will still praise Him,
my Savior and my God."
(Psalm 42:5 hcsb)

Key Passage to Read

Lamentations 3:19–26 (NLT)
"The thought of my suffering . . . is bitter beyond words.
20 I will never forget this awful time, as I grieve over my loss.
21 Yet I still dare to hope when I remember this:
22 The faithful love of the LORD never ends! His mercies never cease.
23 Great is his faithfulness; his mercies begin afresh each morning.
24 I say to myself, 'The LORD is my inheritance; therefore, I will hope in him!'
25 The LORD is good to those who depend on him, to those who search for him.
26 So it is good to wait quietly for salvation from the LORD."

My Personalized Plan to Manage Depression and Live with Hope

Depression can hide the light of day from my view and leave me in the darkness of despair. A sense of hopelessness lingers. But amidst the heaviness and dark clouds of depression, God wants to lift my heavy heart and show me there is hope.

> *"There is surely a future hope for you,*
> *and your hope will not be cut off."*
> (Proverbs 23:18)

Because depression can impact every area of my life, I must address it from multiple angles. As I walk through the darkness of depression into the light of dawn, **I will . . .**

Recognize that my depression is real.
- I will acknowledge my feelings of sadness, anger, hopelessness, and other overwhelming emotions.
- I will not live in denial about my depression but will educate myself about depression and seek help to move forward.

"I am suffering and in pain. Rescue me, O God, by your saving power" (PSALM 69:29 NLT).

Remember that my pain is temporary.
- I will put my pain in perspective and acknowledge that God can help me.
- I will remember that God will one day put an end to all pain and suffering.

"He will wipe every tear from their eyes, and there will be no more death or sorrow or crying or pain. All these things are gone forever" (Revelation 21:4 NLT).

Reaffirm the importance of caring for my physical needs.
- I will talk with my doctor about my depression and get regular medical check-ups.

- I will eat nutritious meals, get adequate sleep each night, and exercise regularly.

"Physical training is of some value, but godliness has value for all things, holding promise for both the present life and the life to come" (1 TIMOTHY 4:8).

Restrict the amount of stress in my life.
- I will identify the environmental or situational factors related to my depression, such as difficult life events,
- losses I've experienced, and the various sources of stress in my life.
- I will seek to adjust to stressful life events and deal with my losses in a healthy, productive manner.

"Give me relief from my distress; have mercy on me and hear my prayer" (PSALM 4:1).

Reveal my emotional needs.
- I will talk with a trusted friend or family member, counselor, and especially with God about my emotions.
- I will honestly confront my feelings and process them with God's help.

"I call to you, LORD, every day; I spread out my hands to you" (PSALM 88:9).

Restrain negative thought patterns.
- I will acknowledge negative self-talk and lies I believe about myself or my situation.
- I will replace negative thoughts with God's truth by meditating on His Word.

"Whatever is true, whatever is noble, whatever is right, whatever is pure, whatever is lovely, whatever is admirable— if anything is excellent or praiseworthy—think about such things" (Philippians 4:8).

Renew my commitment to get my spiritual needs met.
- I will cultivate my relationship with God through reflective prayer and Bible reading.
- I will attend church regularly to receive encouragement from God's Word and to be with other believers.

"All the believers devoted themselves to the apostles' teaching, and to fellowship, and to sharing in meals (Including the Lord's Supper), *and to prayer"* (Acts 2:42 NLT).

How to Help a Depressed Loved One

When you have depressed loved ones in your life, you want to do something that will make a difference, but the question is *what?*

First and foremost, *do not avoid them.* Because of the tendency to withdraw and isolate, help them get involved in activities whenever they are open to doing so. Encourage them to find a new hobby. Realize, you may be their only lifeline of hope, and they need to stay connected. Do what you wish someone would do for you if you were struggling with depression.

> *"Do to others as you would have them do to you."*
> (Luke 6:31)

12 Things You Can Do to Help

Learn all you can about depression.

Read books, watch videos, attend conferences, visit websites such as the National Institute of Mental Health (www.nimh.nih.gov).
"Apply your heart to instruction and your ears to words of knowledge" (Proverbs 23:12).

Be an accountability partner.
Communicate both with words and actions, "I'm with you in this, and I won't abandon you."
"I have no one else like Timothy, who genuinely cares about your welfare" (Philippians 2:20 NLT).

Initiate regular dialogue.
Send frequent text messages and phone calls. Make intentional contact and encourage them sincerely and often.
"Let everything you say be good and helpful, so that your words will be an encouragement to those who hear them" (Ephesians 4:29 NLT).

Listen to their pain.
Take time to hear their story and let them share their feelings without fear of judgment. Listening affirms their value and helps them process their emotions and circumstances.
"Everyone should be quick to listen, slow to speak and slow to become angry" (JAMES 1:19).

Talk about depression
Talking about depression helps remove the stigma of it.
"A word fitly spoken is like apples of gold in a setting of silver" (Proverbs 25:11 esv).

Help them find a support group.
There is strength in numbers. Inquire at a nearby hospital, local church, or search the web for listings of support groups in the community dealing with depression or mental illness.
"Two people are better off than one, for they can help each other succeed. If one person falls, the other can reach out and help" (Ecclesiastes 4:9–10 NLT).

Realize the power of touch.
As appropriate, a hand on the shoulder or a hug can be a great comfort.
"Greet one another with a kiss of love" (1 Peter 5:14).

Play inspirational music when you're with them.
Music is therapeutic and can lift their spirit.
". . . speaking to one another with psalms, hymns and songs from the Spirit" (Ephesians 5:19).

Bring laughter into their lives.
Share funny cards, pictures, stories, videos, or movies.
"A cheerful heart is good medicine" (Proverbs 17:22).

Work with them to set small, daily goals.
Encourage them to set and achieve small goals that require minimal effort. Check on their progress regularly.
"The desires of the diligent are fully satisfied" (Proverbs 13:4).

Enlist help from other family and friends.

DEALING WITH SUICIDE & DEPRESSION

Be specific about your concerns and engage others in caring for the one depressed.
"Carry each other's burdens, and in this way you will fulfill the law of Christ" (Galatians 6:2).

Take all threats of suicide seriously.
If suicide is a concern, ask, "Are you thinking about hurting yourself or taking your life?" While asking this may create some discomfort, awkwardness, or make them initially upset—it is worth the risk. Don't shy away from the hard questions, but always ask them in a kind and gentle way.
"A prudent person foresees danger and takes precautions" (Proverbs 27:12 NLT).

How to Respond to Suicidal Thoughts or Threats

If you, or a depressed loved one, are having suicidal thoughts or planning to harm yourself, it is important to talk with someone immediately. You will find information for the National Suicide Prevention Lifeline and the Crisis Text Line below. These free and confidential services are available 24/7 to provide emotional support and helpful resources for those facing distress and having suicidal thoughts. When you contact them, you will be connected with a real person who is trained to provide guidance and support. You are *not* alone.

> *"Be strong and courageous.*
> *Do not be afraid or terrified . . .*
> *for the LORD your God goes with you;*
> *he will never leave you nor forsake you."*
> (Deuteronomy 31:6)

NOTE: If you are ever in imminent danger, call 911 immediately.

National Suicide Prevention Lifeline
- 1-800-273-TALK (8255)
- 1-800-799-4889 (For Deaf + Hard of Hearing)
- Ayuda disponible en Español
- www.SuicidePreventionLifeline.org (Live chat available)

Crisis Text Line
- Text HOME to 741741 (United States)
- Text HOME to 686868 (Canada)
- Text HOME to 85258 (United Kingdom)
- www.CrisisTextLine.org

Don't hesitate to call or text these hotlines if you're thinking of harming yourself. Remember, no matter what you're feeling or how bad things seem . . .

"There is surely a future hope for you."
(Proverbs 23:18)

Go Deeper

Keys for Living Books

Want to learn more about this topic? Check out the *Keys for Living Library* to discover biblical hope and practical help on this topic and many more. The *Keys for Living* are designed to help you—and help you help others—overcome difficulties, grow in maturity, and move forward in life.

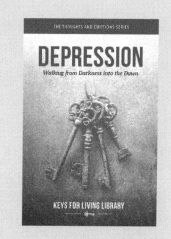

hopefortheheart.org/keys

Topical Video Training

Check out our *Lifeline to Hope* Topical Video Course on this topic. These videos provide biblical insights and practical guidance on specific emotional, relational, and spiritual issues.

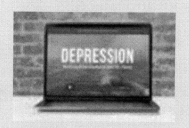

hopefortheheart.org/topical

4 POINTS OF GOD'S PLAN

Whether you're trying to make sense of your past, trying to overcome something in the present, or trying to make changes for a better future, the Lord cares about you. He loves you. No matter what challenges you or your loved ones are facing, no matter the pain or difficult feelings you may be experiencing, no matter what you've done or what's been done to you, *there is hope*. And that hope is found in Jesus Christ.

God has a plan for your life, and it begins with a personal relationship with Jesus. The most important decision you can ever make is whether you will accept His invitation. If you have never made that decision, these four simple truths can help you start your journey together with Him.

> *"'For I know the plans I have for you,' declares the LORD,*
> *'plans to prosper you and not to harm you,*
> *plans to give you hope and a future.'"*
> (Jeremiah 29:11)

God's Purpose for You: *Salvation*

What was God's motivation in sending Jesus Christ to earth? To express His love for you by saving you! The Bible says, *"God so loved the world that he gave his one and only Son, that whoever believes in him shall not perish but have eternal life. For God did not send his Son into the world to condemn the world, but to save the world through him"* (John 3:16–17).

What was Jesus' purpose in coming to earth? To forgive your sins, to empower you to have victory over sin, and to enable you to live a fulfilled life! Jesus said, *"I have come that they may have life, and have it to the full"* (John 10:10).

The Problem: *Sin*

What exactly is sin? Sin is living independently of God's standard—knowing what is wrong and doing it anyway—also knowing what is right and choosing not to do it. The apostle Paul said, *"I know that nothing good lives in me, that is, in my sinful nature. I want to do what is right, but I can't. I want to do what is good, but I don't. I don't want to do what is wrong, but I do it anyway"* (Romans 7:18–19 NLT).

What is the major consequence of sin? Spiritual death, eternal separation from God. The Bible says, *"Your iniquities* [sins] *have separated you from your God"* (Isaiah 59:2). Scripture also says, *"The wages of sin is death, but the gift of God is eternal life in Christ Jesus our Lord"* (Romans 6:23).

God's Provision for You: *The Savior*

Can anything remove the penalty for sin? Yes! Jesus died on the cross to personally pay the penalty for your sins. The Bible says, *"God demonstrates his own love for us in this: While we were still sinners, Christ died for us"* (Romans 5:8).

What is the solution to being separated from God? Belief in (entrusting your life to) Jesus Christ as the only way to God the Father. Jesus said, *"I am the way and the truth and the life. No one comes to the Father except through me"* (John 14:6). The Bible says, *"Believe in the Lord Jesus, and you will be saved . . ."* (Acts 16:31).

Your Part: *Surrender*

Give Christ control of your life, entrusting yourself to Him. Jesus said, *"Whoever wants to be my disciple must deny themselves and take up their cross and follow me. For whoever wants to save their life will lose it, but whoever loses their life for me will find it. What good will it be for someone to gain the whole world, yet forfeit their soul?"* (Matthew 16:24–26).

Place your faith in (rely on) Jesus Christ as your personal Lord and Savior and reject your "good works" as a means of earning God's approval. The Bible says, *"It is by grace you have been saved, through faith—and this is not from yourselves, it is the gift of God—not by works, so that no one can boast"* (Ephesians 2:8–9).

Has there been a time in your life when you know you've humbled your heart and received Jesus Christ as your personal Lord and Savior—giving Him control of your life? You can tell God that you want to surrender your life to Christ in a simple, heartfelt prayer like this:

"God, I want a real relationship with you.
I admit that many times I've chosen to go my own way instead of your way.
Please forgive me for my sins.
Jesus, thank you for dying on the cross to pay the penalty for my sins.
Come into my life to be my Lord and my Savior.
Change me from the inside out and make me
the person you created me to be.
In your holy name I pray. Amen."

What Can You Now Expect?

When you surrender your life to Christ, you receive the Holy Spirit who empowers you to live a life pleasing to God. The Bible says, *"His divine power*

DEALING WITH SUICIDE & DEPRESSION

has given us everything we need for a godly life . . ." (2 Peter 1:3). Jesus assures those who believe with these words:

"Truly I tell you, whoever hears my word and believes him who sent me has eternal life and will not be judged but has crossed over from death to life."
(John 5:24)

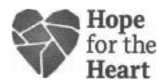

P.O. Box 7, Dallas, TX 75221
hopefortheheart.org

© 2021 Hope for the Heart

The information in this resource is intended as guidelines for healthy living. Please consult qualified medical, legal, pastoral, and psychological professionals regarding individual concerns.

Unless otherwise indicated, all Scripture quotations are taken from The Holy Bible, New International Version®, NIV® Copyright © 1973, 1978, 1984, 2011 by Biblica, Inc.™ Used by permission. All rights reserved worldwide.

Scripture quotations marked (ESV) are taken from The ESV® Bible (The Holy Bible, English Standard Version®), copyright © 2001 by Crossway, a publishing ministry of Good News Publishers. Used by permission. All rights reserved.

Scripture quotations marked (NKJV) are taken from the New King James Version®. Copyright © 1982 by Thomas Nelson, Inc. Used by permission. All rights reserved.

Scripture quotations marked (NLT) are taken from the Holy Bible, New Living Translation, copyright © 1996, 2004, 2015 by Tyndale House Foundation. Used by permission of Tyndale House Publishers, Inc., Carol Stream, Illinois 60188. All rights reserved.

Scripture quotations marked (NASB) are from the New American Standard Bible®, Copyright © 1960, 1962, 1963, 1968, 1971, 1972, 1973, 1975, 1977, 1995 by The Lockman Foundation. Used by permission. (www.Lockman.org)

Scripture quotations marked (HCSB) are taken from the Holman Christian Standard Bible®, Copyright © 1999, 2000, 2002, 2003, 2009 by Holman Bible Publishers. Used by permission. Holman Christian Standard Bible®, Holman CSB®, and HCSB® are federally registered trademarks of Holman Bible Publishers.

QUESTIONS FOR REFLECTION

God gives us His Word not just for information but for transformation. The Lord wants you to *"be transformed by the renewing of your mind"* (Romans 12:2). This isn't something you do alone, but something God does in you by His Spirit.

The following questions are designed to help you reflect on the biblical truths in this resource. Take a moment to pray and ask God to settle your mind and quiet your spirit as you reflect on His truth.

> *"Reflect on what I am saying, for the Lord*
> *will give you insight into all this."*
> (2 Timothy 2:7)

What are two key truths, Bible verses, or "takeaways" from this resource that you found helpful—or that you simply needed to be reminded of?

_____
_____
_____
_____

In relation to this topic, what behavior(s) do you need to *begin, change*, or *stop* in order to help you grow into the person God created you to be?

_____
_____
_____
_____

DEALING WITH SUICIDE & DEPRESSION

In relation to this topic, what is the biggest obstacle you need to overcome in order to move forward?

What might your life look like a few years from now if you do *not* make changes regarding this issue? How might your life be different if you *do* make changes?

Is there anyone in your life who needs help with this topic/issue? How can you pray for them, and what is one thing you can do to encourage them?

What can you give thanks to God for today?

> *"Now may our Lord Jesus Christ himself*
> *and God our Father, who loved us*
> *and by his grace gave us eternal comfort*
> *and a wonderful hope,*
> *comfort you and strengthen you*
> *in every good thing you do and say."*
> (2 Thessalonians 2:16–17 NLT)

DID YOU KNOW ... ?

**You can get any of our *Lifeline to Hope*
Topical Video Courses for 30% off!**

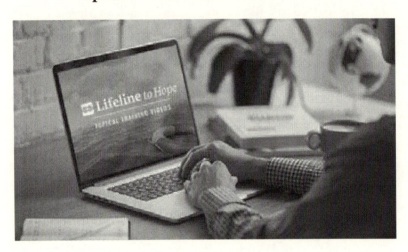

Use code TOPICAL30 at checkout and take 30% off today!

Our topical video courses provide biblical instruction and practical guidance on specific emotional, relational, and spiritual issues such as Abuse, Addiction, Anger, Anxiety, Depression, Fear, Forgiveness, Grief, Marriage, Parenting, Stress, and more. Get the tools to face life's challenges with courage and confidence.

DEALING WITH SUICIDE & DEPRESSION

These video courses are great for:
- Personal study and growth—helping you overcome specific personal challenges
- Learning how to help others move toward greater freedom and spiritual maturity
- Anyone who wants to learn more about what God's Word teaches on various subjects

Each video course includes a downloadable workbook with helpful, biblical insights on the topic and discussion questions for further study and growth.

hopefortheheart.org/topical 20220311

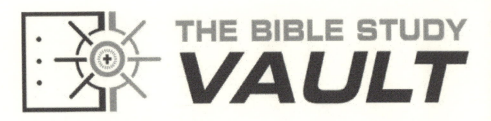

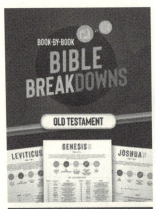 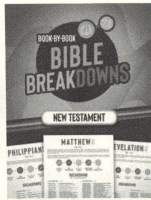 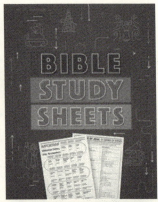

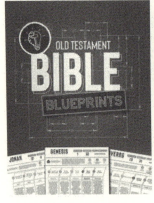 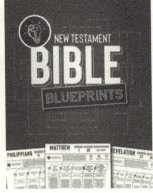 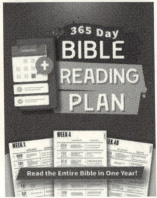

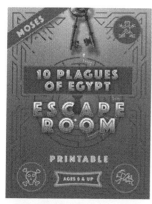
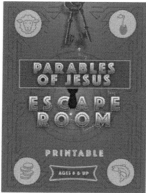
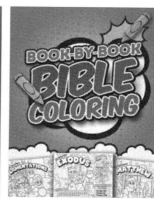
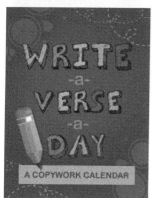
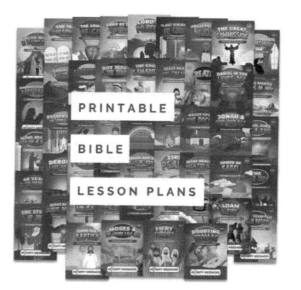

CLICK COVERS
TO LEARN MORE

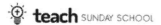

THANK YOU

Thank you for ordering from www.TeachSundaySchool.com. We strive to offer you top notch Bible teaching tools. Feel free to contact us with any questions a **marykate@teachsundayschool.com**.

HOW TO PRINT

If you are having any trouble printing, here are some helpful tips:

1. Adobe Acrobat PDF Reader is the most universal PDF reader and comes standard on most computers. If you are having issues, check to make sure you are using a recent version of Adobe, which is available free online here.
2. If for any reason a page is being cut off, when you push the "print" button and the dialogue box pops up, check the box "fit".

TERMS OF USE

The material enclosed is copyrighted. You do not have resell rights or giveaway rights to the material provided herein. Only customers that have purchased this material are authorized to view it.

Allowed:

You are able to print as many times as you would like for personal, family, or single church/school use. (Please show this to any printer you may take this to in order to prove that you are not infringing on the copyright by printing this file).

If you would like to use this file for multiple schools or churches, please email us at marykate@teachsundayschool.com for information on a bundle purchase price.

Not Allowed:

This digital file cannot be given to anyone else. In order to own a digital file, it must be purchased.

This file is never to be emailed to anyone else for the purpose of giving it to them or sharing it with them. In order to own a file, it must be purchased.

Do not post this file, or images from this file on a blog, website, or anything like it for the purpose of giving it away or selling it.

Do not change this file in any way.

DEALING WITH SUICIDE & DEPRESSION

Do not use all or part of this file for commercial use in any way.

Anything that is not meant for the intended use of this file, which is for personal, family, or single church/school use is not allowed. We are offering this as a digital file for the convenience of our customers. Any abuse of that is not allowed.

If you feel you have obtained an unauthorized copy of this material, please email us at marykate@teachsundayschool.com.

LEGAL NOTICE

While all attempts have been made to verify information provided in this publication, neither the author nor the publisher assumes any responsibility for errors, omissions or contrary interpretation of the subject matter herein. The publisher wants to stress that the information contained herein may be subject to varying state and / or local laws or regulations. All users are advised to retain competent counsel to determine what state and / or local laws or regulations may apply to the user's particular operation.

The purchaser or reader of this publication assumes responsibility for the use of these materials and information. Adherence to all applicable laws and regulations, federal, state and local, governing professional licensing, operation practices, and all other aspects of operation in the US or any other jurisdiction is the sole responsibility of the purchaser or reader. The publisher and author assume no responsibility or liability whatsoever on the behalf of any purchaser or reader of these materials. Any perceived slights of specific people or organizations is unintentional.

THE RETURN OF THE PRODIGAL SON BY HENRI NOUWEN

LUKE 15:11-32

Jesus shows u what true sonship is. He is the younger son without being rebellious.

He is the elder son without being resentful. In everything he is obedient to the Father, but never His slave.

He hears everything the Father says, but this does not make him his servant.

He does everything the Father sends Him to do, but remains completely free.

He gives everything and receives everything.

He declares openly: "In all truth I tell you, by himself the Son can do nothing.

He can only do what He sees the Father doing, and whatever the Father does the Son does too.

For the Father loves the Son and shows him everything he himself does , and he will show Him even greater things than these works that will astonish you.

Thas as the Father raises the dead and gives them life, so the Son gives life to anyone He choses; for the Father judges no one; he has entrusted all judgement to the Son, so that all may honor the Son as they honor the Father.

THE HEART OF GOD

In Rembrandt's painting, the elder son simply observes. It is difficult to imagine what is going on in his heart. How will he respond to the invitation to join the celebration?

There is no doubt-in the parable or the painting-about the Father's heart.

His heart goes out to both of his sons; He loves them both, he hopes to see them together as brothers around the same table; he wants them to experience that, different as they are, they belong to the same household and are children of the same Father.

The story of the Father and his lost sons powerfully affirms that it was not I who chose God, but God who first chose me.

This is the great mystery of our faith. We do not choose God, God choses us.

From all eternity we are hidden "in the shadows of God's hand: and "engraved on His palm.

(insert the picture of the image taken in space of "GOD'S HAND).

Before any human touches us, God "forms us in secret" & "textures us" in the depth of the earth, and before any human being decides about us, God "knits us together in our Mother's womb".

God loves us before any human person can show love to us. He loves us with a "first" love, an unlimited, unconditional love, wants us to be his beloved children, and tells us to become as loving as himself.

Sometimes we wonder whether we have realized that during this time that God has been trying to find me, to know me, and to love me.

The question is not "How am I to find God?" but "How am I to let myself be found by Him?"

The question is not "How am I to know God?" but "How am I to let myself be known by God?"

And finally

The question is not "How am I to love God?" but "How am I to let myself be loved by God?"

Personal statement:

This is the hardest part for me and many others as we do not understand how God could love us especially when we do not love ourselves. I have learned that God's love is not dependent on how we feel about ourselves because if it was then that would mean that the sacrifice on the cross was not enough to close the great divide between us and God.

God is looking into the distance for me, trying to find me, and bring me home.

Personal statement:

Just like in the Garden of Eden when God was looking for Adam and Eve after they partake from the tree of the knowledge of good and evil. Do you really think that God did not know where they were hiding?

Why do we think we can hide from God?

In all three parables in Luke 15 Jesus tells in response to the question of why he eats with sinners, he puts the emphasis of God's initative.

God is the shepherd who goes looking for His lost sheep.

God is the woman who lights a lamp, sweeps out the house, and searches everywhere for her lost coin until she has found it.

God is the Father who watches and waits for His children, runs out to meet them, embraces them,pleads with them, begs and urges them to come home.

It might sound strange, but God wants to find me as much as if not more than I want to find God.

Yes, God needs me as much as I need God.

God is not the patriarch who stays home, doesn't move, and expects His children to come to Him, apologize for their oberrhant behavior, beg for forgiveness and promise to do better.

To the contrary, He leaves the house, ignoring his dignity by running toward them, pays no attention to apologies and promises of change, and brings them to the table richly prepared for them.

For a very long time I considered Low self-esteem to be some kind of virtue. I had been warned against pride so often that I came to consider it a good thing to belittle myself.

But know I realize that the real sin is to deny God's first love for me, to ignore my original goodness.

DEALING WITH SUICIDE & DEPRESSION

Because without claiming that first love and that original goodness for myself, I lose touch with my true self and embark on the destructive search among the wrong people and in the wrong places for what can only be found in the house of my Father.

(Insert the diagram of the 48 prophecies foretold about Jesus in the Old Testament), (teach Sunday School)

MOMENTS WITH GOD: "A lack of clarity is always a call to deeper intimacy"-Vance Pittman

For we are God's masterpiece. He has created us anew in Christ Jesus, so we can do the good things he planned for us long ago. Ephesians 2:10

Following words from a song by Josh Baldwin:

I know who I am because I know who You are-The Cross of Salvation was only the start

Now I am chosen, free and forgiven-I have a future and it's worth the living

Cause I wasn't made to be tending a grave-I was called by name

Born and raised back to life again-I was made for more

So why would I make a bed in my shame-When a fountain of grace is running my way

I know I am yours-And I was made for more

Oh hallelujah -You called out my name

Michael Donald Misfeldt

So I'll sing out your praise-Hallelujah

You buried my past-And I'm not going back

Create in me a pure heart, O God, and renew a steadfast spirit within me. Do not cast me from your presence or take your Holy Spirit from me. Restore to me the joy of your salvation and grant me a willing spirit to sustain me. Psalm 51: 10-12

**Navigators
Discipleship
Tool**

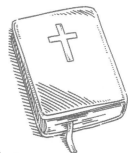

Know Your Identity in Christ:
Bible Verses to Memorize

When you know your identity is in Christ, it will change your outlook on life. Deciding to trust and follow Jesus is the first step of becoming a new person. It's because of His death, burial, and resurrection that you have been made new (2 Corinthians 5:17). However, it's easy to forget who you are in Christ when the world's messages feel much louder than the truth of God's Word.

Here are 26 verses going through each letter of the alphabet to remind you who you are in Christ. Select a handful from this list or even try memorizing all 26 Scripture passages. Consider inviting a friend to join you and see how knowing who you are in Christ changes how you live.

In Christ, you are...

In Christ, you are...

*A*dopted

"he predestined us for adoption to sonship through Jesus Christ, in accordance with his pleasure and will."

Ephesians 1:5 (NIV)

In Christ, you are...

*B*eloved

"Therefore, as God's chosen people, holy and dearly loved, clothe yourselves with compassion, kindness, humility, gentleness and patience."

Colossians 3:12 (NIV)

In Christ, you are...

*C*hosen

"For he chose us in him before the creation of the world to be holy and blameless in his sight."

Ephesians 1:4 (NIV)

In Christ, you are...

*D*elighted In

"The LORD your God is with you, the Mighty Warrior who saves. He will take great delight in you; in his love he will no longer rebuke you, but will rejoice over you with singing."

Zephaniah 3:17 (NIV)

In Christ, you are...

*E*stablished

"Now to him who is able to establish you in accordance with my gospel, the message I proclaim about Jesus Christ, in keeping with the revelation of the mystery hidden for long ages past...."

Romans 16:25 (NIV)

In Christ, you are...

*F*orgiven

"If we confess our sins, he is faithful and just and will forgive us our sins and purify us from all unrighteousness."

1 John 1:9 (NIV)

Navigators Discipleship Tool

In Christ, you are...
Given Everything You Need
"His divine power has given us everything we need for a godly life through our knowledge of him who called us by his own glory and goodness."

2 Peter 1:3 (NIV)

In Christ, you are...
Heir
"Now if we are children, then we are heirs—heirs of God and co-heirs with Christ, if indeed we share in his sufferings in order that we may also share in his glory."

Romans 8:17 (NIV)

In Christ, you are...
Invited
"All those the Father gives me will come to me, and whoever comes to me I will never drive away."

John 6:37 (NIV)

In Christ, you are...
Justified
"Therefore, since we have been justified through faith, we have peace with God through our Lord Jesus Christ...."

Romans 5:1 (NIV)

In Christ, you are...
Known
"You have searched me, LORD, and you know me. You know when I sit and when I rise; you perceive my thoughts from afar."

Psalm 139:1-2 (NIV)

In Christ, you are...
Loved
"This is love: not that we loved God, but that he loved us and sent his Son as an atoning sacrifice for our sins."

1 John 4:10 (NIV)

In Christ, you are...
Masterpiece
"For we are God's handiwork, created in Christ Jesus to do good works, which God prepared in advance for us to do."

Ephesians 2:10 (NIV)

In Christ, you are...
Not Condemned
"Therefore, there is now no condemnation for those who are in Christ Jesus."

Romans 8:1 (NIV)

In Christ, you are...
Oak of Righteousness
"They will be called oaks of righteousness, a planting of the LORD for the display of his splendor."

Isaiah 61:3b (NIV)

In Christ, you are...
Purified
"...let us draw near to God with a sincere heart and with the full assurance that faith brings, having our hearts sprinkled to cleanse us from a guilty conscience and having our bodies washed with pure water."

Hebrews 10:22 (NIV)

DEALING WITH SUICIDE & DEPRESSION

 Navigators Discipleship Tool

In Christ, you are...
Qualified
"Such confidence we have through Christ before God. Not that we are competent in ourselves to claim anything for ourselves, but our competence comes from God. He has made us competent as ministers of a new covenant—not of the letter but of the Spirit; for the letter kills, but the Spirit gives life." 2 Corinthians 3:4-6 (NIV)

In Christ, you are...
Redeemed
"It is because of him that you are in Christ Jesus, who has become for us wisdom from God—that is, our righteousness, holiness and redemption."
1 Corinthians 1:30 (NIV)

In Christ, you are...
Sustained
"Cast your cares on the LORD and he will sustain you; he will never let the righteous be shaken."
Psalm 55:22 (NIV)

In Christ, you are...
Treasured
"But you are a chosen people, a royal priesthood, a holy nation, God's special possession, that you may declare the praises of him who called you out of darkness into his wonderful light."
1 Peter 2:9 (NIV)

In Christ, you are...
Unashamed
"As Scripture says, 'Anyone who believes in him will never be put to shame.'"
Romans 10:11 (NIV)

In Christ, you are...
Victorious
"But thanks be to God! He gives us the victory through our Lord Jesus Christ."
1 Corinthians 15:57 (NIV)

In Christ, you are...
Welcomed
"In him and through faith in him we may approach God with freedom and confidence."
Ephesians 3:12 (NIV)

In Christ, you are...
EXquisitely Made
"For you created my inmost being; you knit me together in my mother's womb."
Psalm 139:13 (NIV)

In Christ, you are...
Lightly Yoked
"'Come to me, all you who are weary and burdened, and I will give you rest. Take my yoke upon you and learn from me, for I am gentle and humble in heart, and you will find rest for your souls. For my yoke is easy and my burden is light.'"
Matthew 11:28-30 (NIV)

In Christ, you are...
One Whom God is Zealous For
"But because of his great love for us, God, who is rich in mercy, made us alive with Christ even when we were dead in transgressions—it is by grace you have been saved."
Ephesians 2:4-5 (NIV)

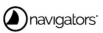

THIS TOOL IS MEANT TO BE SHARED. **To download a copy, visit navlink.org/identity**

I am a Child of God

I'm not a preacher or an evangelist, but what I am is a Child of God. And when you truly recognize that, you start to see your purpose in this journey called life: to share the Gospel with the people you love and those God has placed in your life. It's a calling that's both beautiful and, yes, sometimes a little scary. Why? Because we're afraid that if we share the Gospel, people might not like us anymore—or even worse, reject us. That fear is natural, and it doesn't mean you're a bad Christian for feeling it.

Even Jesus wasn't fully accepted in His own hometown, but that didn't stop Him from preaching truth—always in love. And that's key. If we don't share the Gospel with those we love, we're not even giving them the chance to accept or reject it. That's not what we're called to do.

But I hear you—"What if I don't know what to say? What if I mess it up?" It's not about getting the message perfectly right. God has already given us the message: We've all sinned, and to be right with a holy God, we need to repent and ask for forgiveness. Jesus has already paid the price, and all we need to do is accept His grace. That's it. You don't have to worry about delivering it flawlessly—just speak from the heart and let God do the rest.

1. **Truth about God**: His grace is not dependent on our willingness to accept it. *Let that sink in*—His grace is not conditional on us. (repeat 2X). His forgiveness comes when we admit our sin, but His grace? It's a constant, always available, no matter how we respond.

2. **Truth about God**: God has chosen you to show His love to those around you, especially your loved ones. Their acceptance or rejection of that love doesn't determine its power. And guess what? They might not respond positively right away—and that's OKAY! Our God is so patient. He will give them many opportunities because His love is infinite. He loves His children far beyond what we can even imagine—more than we could ever love our own children. What parent doesn't want the best for their kids?

3. **Truth about God**: Anything you place before God will eventually disappoint you. I learned this the hard way. I used to love my work so much that it became an idol, more important than my family and even God. I was proud of my achievements and reputation, and honestly, I was a workaholic. But over time, God—patient and loving—showed me that even though I idolized my work, He was still there, guiding me through every season. After 40 years in the trucking industry, I can now see that God has always been preparing me for each step, even when I felt overlooked or treated unfairly. He never left me, even when my trust in Him wavered.

4. **Truth about God**: He uses our weaknesses to strengthen our faith. For a long time, I was afraid to talk about Jesus. Why? Because I was scared of what people would think. But here's the truth—why should I worship the idol of fear? For too long, I did just that. And God, in His mercy, showed me that fear was never meant to be worshipped. He reminded me that He is faithful, even when I was on disability and feared I wouldn't return to work. He never let me down.

5. **Truth about God**: His plans are so much better than ours. Think about why you're here, now, reading this—maybe it's because you're seeking something deeper. Maybe you're ready to follow Jesus and walk the path He's laid out for you. But what's stopping you? Is it a lack of trust? Is it feelings of inadequacy? Whatever it is, God's already taken care of it. It's not about you or me—it's about responding to the call as a Child of God.

This is life and death for the people we love. The enemy wants to steal, kill, and destroy (John 10:10), but Jesus came so we could have life to the fullest.

6. In Him is life, the very light of man (John 1:3). God gives us living water through Jesus, but sometimes we turn to broken cisterns—idols that hold nothing. Like it says in Jeremiah 2:13, God's people committed two sins: they turned away from Him, the source of living water, and dug their own broken cisterns that couldn't hold anything. The truth is, idols will always fail us, but God? He offers abundant, unfailing life.

Epilogue

As I reflect on the winding roads of my journey, filled with both trials and triumphs, I recognize the thread of grace that has woven through every chapter of my life. My battles with depression, loss, and self-worth have often clouded my view, but I have come to understand that these moments do not define me—they refine me.

There is no perfect ending to this story, for it is still being written. Each day brings new challenges and new opportunities to grow in faith, in love, and in understanding. But what I have learned is that I am never alone. Whether in the darkest hours of despair or in the light of healing, God's presence is unwavering, His love unconditional.

To anyone reading this, know that no matter the weight of the burdens you carry, there is hope. There is a way forward, even when the path is obscured. Healing is possible, and life—no matter how fractured it may seem—has infinite value.

As I continue on this journey, I embrace the future with an open heart, trusting that there are better days ahead, not because life will always be easy, but because I now understand that I am equipped to face whatever may come.

The journey is not over, but I am ready for whatever comes next.

- **Michael Misfeldt**

Made in the USA
Middletown, DE
04 February 2025